My Yoga Time

This booklet accompanies the My Yoga Time Volume 1 classes and specifically discusses those asanas (poses) practiced. The first part of the booklet details the physical benefits of the asanas and also provides guidance on alignment.

The second part of the book investigates the subtle (energetic) body, prana, and metaphysics. These concepts are thousands of years old, originating in yogic traditions of Hinduism and Buddhism. Please note that yoga is not a religion; many people in the Western world are drawn to yoga for its physical and therapeutic attributes. Should any yogic philosophy not resonate with you, then simply let it go and focus on what does resonate.

CONTENTS

Introduction

The intention of this book and DVD combination is to enhance your understanding of what's happening on all levels in your body and mind throughout your Hatha yoga practice. Yoga has been practiced for over five thousand years, originating in India, and is taught and studied as a science for personal evolution.

This manual is a guide; it does not discuss the history, evolution, or the eight limbs of Ashtanga yoga. This handbook focuses on Hatha yoga, which comprises the third limb, asana (physical poses), and the fourth limb, pranayama (regulation / control of prana through the breath). Although this book briefly discusses pranayama, it does not delve into the study and devoted practice of the fourth limb. Hatha yoga is thought to be the most popular form of yoga in the West because the physical practice eliminates distractions from the mind by *first* stilling the body. Over time, this enhances the mind-body awareness, and cultivates the subtle sensations within and without. At its heart though, Hatha yoga is more than flexibility and strength; it is the management of prana, the vital life-force energy that resides in all life forms: humans, animals, and plants.

The intention of this book is to help bridge the gap between the physical, metaphysical, and spiritual. As your practice evolves, I encourage you to journal your experiences, reference this book, and be open to learning from your higher self. You will learn more from your personal experience on the mat than you will from reading. I offer my experiences merely as a guide, providing another tool to help *your* practice evolve. Thank you for letting me be of service.

The word yoga translates to 'Yoking'—uniting the mind and body. The physical and mental union is, however, phase one. Through dedication and regular practice, the light shines brighter, the sheaths fall away, and you become phase two: the union between the self and the higher consciousness.

Part One

Sun Salutation (Surya Namaskara)

Sun Salutation may be interpreted as vinyasa (asana-linked breath), a graceful sequence of postures continuously flowing with the breath. It promotes flexibility in the body and is an effective way to physically stretch, tone, and massage the muscles, joints, and internal organs. It also generates prana, the subtle energy that stimulates the psychic body. Physically, it strengthens the back and helps to balance all of the systems in the body (digestive, reproductive, respiratory, and circulatory). Breathing deeply and rhythmically while synchronizing with the body's movements increases mental clarity by bringing fresh oxygenated blood to the brain.

For many yogis, Surya Namaskara is practiced in honor of our inner light.

Mula Bandha

Note: There are many bandhas, though the three main bandhas in Hatha yoga are Mula Bandha, Uddiyana Bandha, and Jalandara Bandha. Bandhas are essentially energy locks, and have a profound effect over one's physical and subtle bodies. For the purpose of this booklet and corresponding practice, we are working only with Mula Bandha.

Mula Bandha offers many physical, mental, and spiritual benefits. Physically, this bandha stimulates and tones the pelvic nerves, and the uro-genital and excretory systems. Applying this bandha during asana practice helps to improve core strength, offering stability, increasing endurance, and protects the lower back. Energetically, this bandha contains the prana (life-force energy) in the body, preventing it from escaping, which enhances the subtle awareness of the relationship between the physical and psychic bodies. As one's practice evolves, effort and energy are used more efficiently. With regular practice, one's energy and vitality increase while mental clarity improves. Subtly, it is understood that Mula Bandha helps to realign the physical, mental, and psychic bodies.

When first practicing Mula Bandha, the initial action / sensation for women is to contract the pelvic floor muscles, and for men to squeeze the perineum muscle – the muscles in between the anus and testes. <u>This bandha should not be practiced by women when they are menstruating.</u> However as one's practice progresses, the sensation of Mula Bandha is also felt a little higher around the pelvic girdle. Still an upward lift although in time this can be isolated from squeezing the pelvic floor alone. Be careful not to clench these muscles repetitively without the awareness of the upward lift, as this could advance to an energetic blockage as opposed to being an energetic lock.   The upward lift rises towards the navel, where it can meet Uddiyana Bandha should that bandha be engaged also. The spiritual awareness with Mula Bandha is associated with the Root Chakra (also the ascension of Shakti energy).

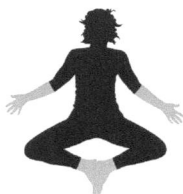

Reclined Butterfly (Supta Baddhakonasana)
-   Opens and stretches the hips, inner thighs, and groin
-   Stretches the knees
-   A restorative pose which allows one to connect with the breath and quiet the mind
-   Increases vitality in the digestive organs, freeing the energy flow in the pelvic region
-   Spiritual awareness: Root and Sacral Chakras
-   *Tip: Slide the shoulder blades back and down the spine. Relax the thighs and groin, and soften through the lower back. Begin to notice the in-breath and the out-breath. This is a wonderful pose to begin any class in, or to meditate and rejuvenate in*

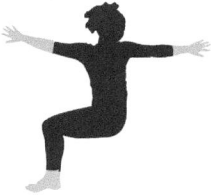

Reclined Twist (Jathara Parivrtti)

- Gently warms the spine and stimulates the digestive organs, kidneys, and liver
- Stretches the back, shoulders, hips, and neck
- Twists lengthen the oblique muscles and the intercostal muscles (mid-section of the body / abdominals)
- Twists in general are therapeutic for menstrual discomforts and sciatica
- Stimulates digestion, aiding in toxin elimination
- Metaphysically, the virtue of a twist is that it wrings stress and tension out of the body as though you are wringing out a sponge
- Spiritual awareness: Solar Plexus Chakra
- *Tip: Apply Mula Bandha on the inhalation to help tone the pelvic floor and energetically stimulate the kundalini energy. Breathe into the lower back when relaxing into the twist.*

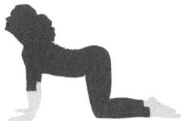

Cat Stretch

- Warms the spine by flexing both front and back sides of the body
- Cat stretch tones the uterus and is therapeutic for menstrual discomfort and after childbirth
- Spiritual awareness: Root and Heart Chakras
- *Tip: Apply Mula Bandha when moving with the breath (either on the inhalation or the exhalation). Maintain downward pressure through the pads of the fingers and knuckles throughout the spinal flexion.*

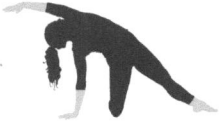

Gate (Parighasana)

- Relaxes the nervous system
- Stimulates the respiratory system
- Lengthens and stretches the entire side of the waist (oblique, intercostals, and latissimus dorsi)
- Opens the chest and hips
- Stretches the ankle and the outside of foot
- Spiritual awareness: Sacral Chakra, and Throat Chakra if maintaining throat lock (Jalandara Bandha)
- *Tip: Stretch the foot of the lengthened leg away from the outreaching arm. Relax the buttocks, and push the hip of the bent leg forward while drawing the hip of the straight leg back. Draw the chin toward the shoulder to lengthen the back of the neck, and support the head (don't let the head drop back).*

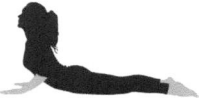

Cobra (Bhujangasana)

- Strengthens the muscles along the spine, increasing flexibility
- Stretches the abdomen, chest, and shoulders
- Stimulates the kidneys and adrenal glands
- Firms the buttocks
- Is therapeutic for fatigue, stress, and respiratory ailments
- Spiritual awareness: Heart Chakra
- *Tip Keep the legs and feet engaged. Push the tops of the feet down, from the little toe to the big toe; lengthen the tailbone down, and push down through the legs to support the back. Energetically draw the hands back while pulling the heart forward, and relax the shoulders away from the ears.*

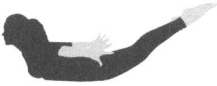

Locust (Shalabasana)

- Strengthens the lower back, shoulders, and legs
- Tones the buttocks
- Stretches the shoulders and thighs
- Stimulates digestion
- Promotes balanced functioning of the bowels, liver, and stomach
- Is therapeutic for fatigue, constipation, and lower back pain
- Spiritual awareness: Sacral & Solar Plexus Chakras
- *Tip Slide the shoulder blades back and down the spine while actively reaching the fingertips away. Extend from the inner thighs through to the big toes, and keep the back of the neck soft. Do not allow the legs to widen as this will put too much pressure on the lumbar spine.*

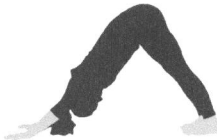

Downward-Facing Dog (Adho Mukha Svanasana)

- Strengthens the legs, arms, and joints
- Stretches the spine, legs, shoulders, calves, and Achilles tendons
- Releases tension in the calf muscles, shoulders, and hips
- Increases the blood circulation throughout the body, especially to the brain, lungs, and various vital organs
- Promotes vitality, relieves tiredness, and rejuvenates the body
- Spiritual awareness: Crown Chakra, and also the Root Chakra through activation of the feet
- *Tip Spread the fingers wide and flatten the palms and fingers, pushing the pads of the fingers into the mat. Relax the head and neck, and roll the shoulder blades back and down the spine. Curl the tail bone up, separating the sit bones while subtly turning the inner thighs in; the heels will gently flare outward so the*

outside edges of feet become parallel to the mat; the inner thighs then engage. Eventually the heels will touch the floor as you push the heart toward the thighs.

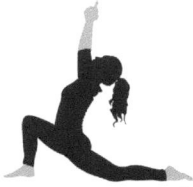

Low Lunge (Ashwa Sanchalanasana)
- Stretches the hip flexors, lower back, and the front knee
- Opens the hips and groin
- Tones the abdominal organs
- Improves sense of balance, also inducing a balanced nervous system
- Spiritual awareness: Sacral Chakra
- *Tip: Activate the thighs by squeezing them toward one another, toward the midline to help support your balance, and avoid putting too much pressure on the lower back. Lengthen the tailbone down.*

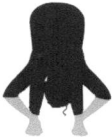

Forward Bend (Uttanasana)
- Stretches the legs, particularly the hamstrings, and back
- Improves sense of balance
- Massages internal organs and increases the blood circulation to the brain
- Calms the brain and is therapeutic for anxiety
- Spiritual awareness: Crown Chakra
- *Tip: Lift and lengthen the toes, then soften the knees slightly; as you inhale, elongate the spine by bringing the heart forward slightly and curling the tailbone up, thighs turning in so the sit bones separate and lift the knees; then as you exhale, hinge*

further forward from the hips, bring more weight to the balls of the feet, then relax the neck and soften the jaw.

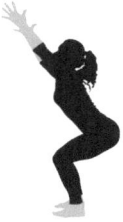

Chair (Utkatasana)

- Stretches the calves, buttocks, and shoulders
- Strengthens the quadriceps, ankles, spine, and shoulders and tones the arms
- Increases core strength
- Is therapeutic for flat feet
- Stimulates the abdominal organs, diaphragm, and heart
- Spiritual awareness: Root Chakra
- *Tip: To protect the knees, do not rotate the hips outward and draw the knees behind the toes. Reaching the arms up, turn the biceps in, and extend the fingers while moving the shoulders away from the ears. Lift and draw the stomach up toward the ribs and lengthen the tailbone down. If the back rounds while the arms are extended, lower them a little so that the back is in one straight line. Keep the groin relaxed.*

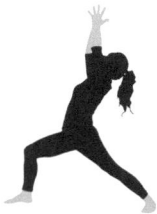

Warrior 1 (Virabradrasana I)

- Stretches, strengthens, and tones the entire body
- Lengthens the psoas muscle (often a difficult muscle to stretch— the important muscle that attaches the legs to the spine)
- Stretches the chest and lungs, shoulders and neck, abdominal organs, groin (psoas), thighs, calves, and ankles

- Strengthens the shoulders, ankles, legs, arms, and the muscles of the back
- Tones and strengthens the abdominal muscles
- Improves balance and posture; also helps to improve concentration, overall circulation, and respiration
- Spiritual awareness Root & Solar Plexus Chakras
- *Tip: Rotate the back thigh in and the front thigh out to assist in opening the hips, then draw the hip of the bent leg back and the hip of the straight leg forward, and lengthen the tailbone down. Lift the arch of the foot on the back straight leg and engage the knee. If there is any pain in the knee, hip, or ankle, lift the back heel off the floor.*

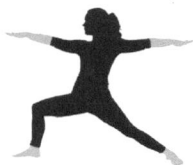

Warrior 2 (Virabradrasana II)
- Strengthens and stretches the legs, ankles, lungs, chest, and shoulders
- Stimulates the abdominal organs
- Is therapeutic for carpel tunnel, flat feet, sciatica, and fatigue
- Spiritual awareness: Sacral Chakra
- *Tip: Direct the front knee over the second toe and look to see the big toe on the inside of the knee, opening up through the hips; lift the arch of the back foot, extending the outside of the foot down and engaging the knee. Rotate the back thigh in and lengthen the tailbone down, drawing the navel in. Hug the feet toward one another, and feel the thighs engage a little more. Roll the shoulders back and down, and soften the upper body.*

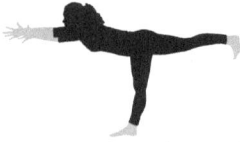

Warrior 3 (Virabradrasana III)

- Strengthens the ankle and knee of the standing leg, shoulders, spine, posterior shoulder muscles, hips, and legs
- Improves stamina and endurance
- Strengthens abdominal muscles
- Helps to develop muscle coordination and concentration, especially through practicing the transition from Virabradrasana I into III
- Spiritual awareness: Sacral & Third Eye Chakras
- *Tip: Rotate the thigh of the lifted leg in; feel as though the thighs are squeezing toward one another. Square the hips and draw the navel up toward the spine.*

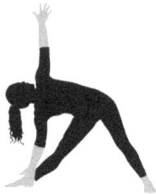

Triangle Pose (Trikonasana)

- Tones the hips and thighs
- Balances the nervous system, and the yin and yang energy within the body
- Promotes a flexible spine
- Opens and stretches the entire side of the body, spine, chest, and hamstrings
- Stretches and strengthens knees and ankles
- Is therapeutic for tension, stress, sciatica, flat feet, and poor posture
- Spiritual awareness: Solar Plexus Chakra, and Throat Chakra when Jalandhara Bandha is applied. Also, through the lengthening of the spine, prana flows more freely and efficiently through sushumna (central nadi)

- *Tip: Lift and engage the front kneecap and thigh; however, if there is a tendency to hyperextend the legs, bring a micro bend to the front knee. If the neck is sore, look down toward the front toe; otherwise, gaze at the top fingers and keep the chin drawn in and the back of the neck long, so the head is not hanging. Keep the fingers on the top hand active to keep the prana from escaping. As you deepen the breath, guide it into the sides of the lungs; feel the spine lengthen, then gently rotate the front-leg hip forward and roll the top hip and shoulder back. Align the shoulders directly above one another.*

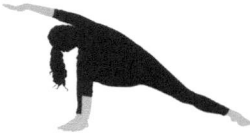

Side Angle Pose (Pasvakonasana)
- Stimulates digestion
- Is therapeutic for constipation, mild low back pain, and menstrual discomfort
- Tones the hips and thighs
- Spiritual Awareness: Solar Plexus Chakra
- *Tip: Ground down the little toe of the straight leg, squeeze the thighs toward one another to engage muscle energy to find additional strength. Gently roll the top hip back to assist the hips in opening and tuck the tailbone under. Actively reach the fingertips of the top hand away from the outside edge of the back foot, and move the chest up and back.*

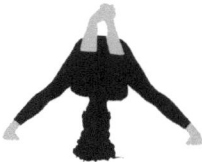

Wide-Leg Forward Bend (Prasarita Padottasana)
- Works the entire back and inside of the legs, from the neck up to the back, and from buttocks down to the knees and ankles

- Is therapeutic for headaches, mild backache, mild depression, and fatigue
- Tones the abdominal organs
- Spiritual Awareness: Crown Chakra
- *Tip: keep the knee caps lifted while gently rotating the inner thighs in so that the sit bones broaden.*

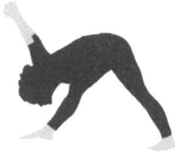

Pyramid (Parsvottanasana)
- Stretches and strengthens the hamstrings
- Improves sense of balance
- Apply Mula Bandha to articulate the sit bones; accentuate this by curling the tailbone up towards the sky
- Spiritual awareness: Root, Solar Plexus, and Throat Chakras
- *Tip: On the inhalation, draw up the arch of the front foot, lift the knee, and engage the thigh, drawing the inner thigh and front hip back, and the back hip forward. Ground down through the outside edge of the back foot and lift the arch. If there is too much pressure behind the front knee, microbend the knee while still keeping the thigh engaged. Inhale and lengthen the spine; bring the heart forward and separate the sit bones; exhale and fold deeper into the pose from the hips, keeping the spine long.*

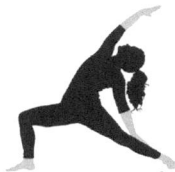

Dancing Warrior (Nataraja Virabrahasana)
- Strengthens the legs, back, knees, and ankles
- Tones and stretches the waistline
- Spiritual awareness: Solar Plexus and Throat Chakras

- *Tip: Turn the bicep of the top arm in to tone and strengthen the arms. Hug the feet toward one another, then continue to sink the down into the lunge as you extend the back, creating space between the ribs.*

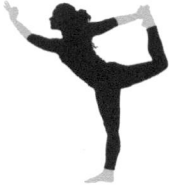

Easy Dancer (Natarajasana)

- Stretches the quadriceps, chest, abdominal psoas muscles, hamstrings, calves, and shoulders
- Opens the lungs
- Strengthens the muscles along the spine, and the knee and ankle of the standing leg
- Balance poses are said to balance the left and right hemispheres of the brain, balancing the nervous system
- Offers relief from a scattered mind, bringing about centeredness and focus
- Improves balance, coordination, and concentration
- Spiritual Awareness: Heart and Third Eye Chakras
- *Tip: Take hold of the foot, before you extend the leg back and upward curl the tailbone up so that the thighs roll in, then tuck the tailbone under allowing a lift and lengthening in the lower back.*

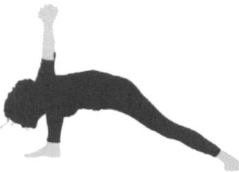

Head to Toe (Sirsha Angustha Yogasana)

- Stretches the hamstring, thighs, and shoulders, and offers a lateral stretch to the body
- Stimulates the nervous system

- Aids in weight reduction around the mid-center
- Strengthens the legs
- Opens the hips
- Spiritual awareness: Sacral Chakra
- *Tip: Draw the front hip back and the back hip forward; take the navel toward the spine and ground down through the outside edge of the back foot.*

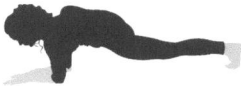

Lizard (Utthan Pristhansana)

- Opens and increases flexibility through the hips and groin
- Strengthens and stretches the legs (particularly the hamstrings and thighs)
- Relieves tension in the hips
- Spiritual awareness: Sacral Chakra
- *Tip: Draw the front hip back and the back hip forward: take the navel toward the spine.*

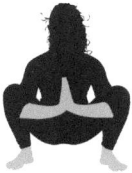

Squat (Malasana or Garland)
- Promotes flexibility in the hips and tones the pelvic floor
- Stretches and strengthens the thighs, knees, ankles, shoulders, buttocks, and neck
- Loosens the pelvic girdle
- Spiritual awareness: Root Chakra

- *Tip: Gently push the elbows into the knees and lift up from the waist to the crown of the head, lengthening the spine.*

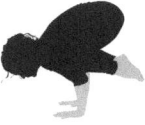

Crow (Bakasana)
- Balances the nervous system
- Strengthens the wrists, shoulders, and arms
- Stretches the upper back and shoulders
- Tones abdominal muscles and improves core strength
- Is said to assist in overcoming the sense of fear
- Spiritual awareness: Root and Third Eye Chakras
- *Tip: Apply Mula Bandha, and squeeze the hands and arms towards one another.*

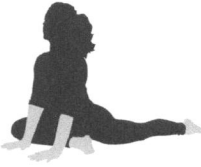

Pigeon (Eka Pada Rajakapotasana)
- Opens the hips and groin
- Is therapeutic for lower back pain and sciatica
- Stretches the buttocks, thighs, knees, and back
- Calms the nervous system
- Spiritual awareness: Root and Sacral Chakras, also the Heart Chakra if practicing the back bend variation
- *Tip: Engage the foot of the bent leg to protect the knee (arch the foot, pushing the top and outside edge of the foot into the mat). Lengthen the tailbone downward.*

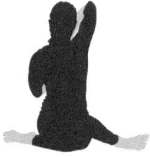

Cow Face (Gomukhasana)

- Opens the hips and lungs
- Stretches the sciatic nerve, hamstring, buttocks, shoulders, and arms
- Improves posture
- Relieves back pain and sciatica
- Is therapeutic for anxiety and tension
- Spiritual awareness: Heart and Third Eye Chakras
- *Tip: As a counter stretch for the shoulders, bring them into Eagle arms (Garudasana arms) after you release your hands.*

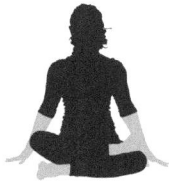

Fire Log (Agnistambhasana)

- Stretches the back and hips, particularly the outer hips, and the groin
- Is therapeutic for stress and sciatica
- Spiritual awareness: Sacral Chakra
- *Tip: Maintain flexion in the feet to protect the knees.*

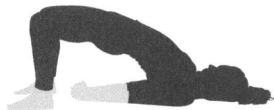

Bridge (Setu Bandhasana)

- Strengthens the muscles along the back
- Lengthens the digestive organs, thus stimulating digestion
- Stretches the quadriceps, shoulders, chest, and lower back

- Relaxes the nervous system and calms the brain
- Stimulates abdominal organs and the thyroid gland
- Is therapeutic for lower back pain, headache, menstrual discomfort, depression, constipation, and respiratory aliments
- Spiritual awareness Heart and Throat Chakras
- *Tip: Turn the toes slightly in so they are closer than the heels to prevent the knees from falling out wide. Avoid jamming the back of the neck; lengthen the neck and move the sternum toward the chin.*

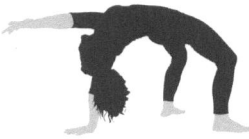

Wild Thing (Camatkarasana)

- Strengthens the wrists, shoulders, and legs
- Opens lungs and shoulders
- Stretches the hip flexors and psoas muscle
- Is therapeutic for fatigue and mild depression
- Spiritual Awareness: Heart Chakra
- *Tip: Draw the top armpit back while simultaneously rolling the shoulder back then ground down through the feet and curl back.*

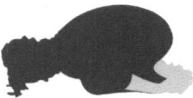

Child's Pose (Balasana)

- Relieves back, shoulder, neck, and hip strain
- Induces a great sense of physical, emotional, and mental relief
- Lengthens the spine
- Balances circulation in the body
- Spiritual Awareness: Root and Third Eye Chakras
- *Tip: Take the knees wide, but keep the big toes touching and sink down a little lower, giving in to gravity.*

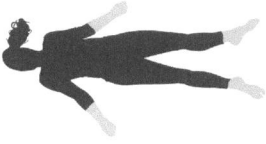

Corpse Pose (Savasana)

Ultimately the most important asana, where the benefits from the practice are truly reaped. The prana pervades the entire body as the nervous system and muscles relax, the mind quiets, and the emotions settle. The body assimilates the prana from the practice, which gently pulsates through the body like ripples on a pond.

- Therapeutic for all stress-related disorders, mild depression, anxiety, fatigue, and insomnia
- Spiritual Awareness: All the Chakras

Part Two

Going Deeper

Yogis believe that the mind and body are not separate entities. Both harbor tension, stress, and dis-ease. It is considered that each mental knot has a corresponding physical knot, and each physical, muscular knot has a corresponding mental or emotional knot / imbalance. The body, as the physical form, is the reflection of the mind and the mind is the subtle form of the body.

Your body will comply with your holistic environment, which comprises both the internal (mental) environment and the external environment. True consciousness doesn't change; the Physical experience and the body is where the change occurs. Consider your body to be a mirror of your internal afflictions. Every thought, every experience is remembered in the body on a cellular level. For thousands of years, yogis have recognized that Hatha yoga is an efficient way to process and release that which is stored in the physical body, and also in the mind, which is no longer serving for your highest good. Each person internalizes his or her experiences and imbalances differently however, so we cannot say that one person's pain in a particular area is going to be similar for everyone. However, certain asanas are said to be effective in releasing emotions and balancing one's state of mind.

Yoga therapy incorporates waste removal and detoxification whether that be purging through the breath, sweating through the pores, or stimulating digestion, and alleviating toxins and constipation. The majority of people do not breathe to the full capacity of their lungs, thus not allowing full expulsion of wastes and carbon dioxide. Often we do not digest efficiently enough to remove all the waste and toxins we ingest. Physically, yoga aids in the digestion and elimination process. There are three types of muscles: skeletal (which move voluntary such as your arms and legs) (arms, legs), cardiac (the heart which moves/ involuntary), and visceral (being the hollow organs and blood vessels, also function/ involuntary. The visceral muscles are transporter muscles (e.g.

intestines) which are not under conscious control. These muscles, along with the cardiac muscles, require certain physical positions (asana), combined with deep breathing techniques (pranaymana) and internal activation (bandhas) for stimulation, thus leading to more active functioning. The visceral muscles are said to hold our deeper primitive emotions, some of our earliest beliefs about ourselves. If muscles do not receive constant messages from the nerves, they deteriorate. This is evidenced in the natural forms of aging. Yoga offers continuous counter-stretching and stimulation (pranic stimulation also), for both the "external" skeletal / voluntary muscles and the cardiac and visceral / involuntary muscles.

Hatha yoga, in particular asana and pranayama, help one to cultivate and sharpen the mind Body awareness and the finer subtle sensations of prana, thus the mind, body, and spirit connect consciously. Through practice and dedication, one learns to direct the prana, the life force energy to where it's needed most in the body. Consider that every time you come to the mat, you are physically processing the emotional and mental afflictions from the day / week /month before, shedding the layers like snake skin. Yoga is more than just mat time. The mat is a place of dedication, appreciation, and self-realization. The body has a limitless sense to heal / expand / change from the subtle level first, the pinnacle from which your life as you know it now, evolves. By consciously influencing the subtle level first, one's selfless intentions / dreams / goals manifest much quicker—first in the mind, then flowing through to your body, and finally your life experiences.

We exist in a world of polarity. Everything, including emotions, has an inevitable polar opposite: nature's seasons, the sun and moon, masculinity / femininity, feelings of bliss and despair—the pendulum swings from one to the other. Through dedicated practice, balance is brought to the mind and body. Where inner peace and happiness is found in the present moment, it is found internally, not through external means. On a subtle level, the mind releases baggage through stilling the body first. Then the mind eventually becomes more centered and remains in the present moment for longer periods of time, allowing one to become the observer, not the thinker, and therefore to be completely present. When one remains present for longer periods of time, it is possible to stay centered and observe the emotional and mental fluctuations without any attachment and unconscious reaction.

When you come to the mat consciously, you begin a beautiful process of self-enquiry. When tuning into the body and feeling it consciously, either on or off the mat, consider any imbalances or afflictions, acknowledge the attachment and the corresponding body part (where this intuitively resonates), and breathe. Direct the breath and therefore the prana into the corresponding body part or chakra, while moving through the appropriate asanas which stimulate this area of the body. By becoming aware of our afflictions, we minimize the risk of being victim to them. When emotions arise during your practice, do not analyze them or form further attachment. By simply acknowledging their presence, one sheds light where there is darkness and an emotional release will follow. A state of calm is regained through breathing consciously.

Asanas are essentially triggers for emotional release. While everyone internalizes his or her experiences differently, certain types of asanas can have a big influence. By recognizing the relationship between metaphysical and anatomical in your practice, you may find the correlation between the physical ailments below and the mental / emotional afflictions. *Refer also to the Chakra chart, where imbalances are compared to the anatomical position of the ailment.*

Asanas / The Body	Metaphysical Release / Emotional Source
Backward Bending Asanas	Associated with embracing life and releasing fears. Backbends open the heart center, physically stimulating the lungs, heart, and back, while subtly opening to grace, light, and love, being the polar opposites of fear and depression. These asanas are invigorating, generating energy and compassion.
Forward Bending Asanas	Metaphysically, forward bends are associated with moving forward in life. It is common for people to force the body in forward bends. Softening in forward bends, giving in to gravity, and being patient with the body will ensure that these positions are more pleasurable. Forward bends encourage one to release the ego and surrender, bringing about a calm state of mind.
Twisting Asanas	The virtue of a twist is that it wrings excess tension and stress out of the body, as though you are wringing out a sponge. Relieves the body of built-up tension.
Inverted Asanas	Inversions often stir up fear, revealing behavioral attitudes, and reluctance to look at one's self and life from a different angle. Inversions literally turn one's world upside down which, when achieved, brings an abundance of confidence as practitioners realize they can support themselves in times of turmoil.
Back Ailments	Generally speaking, the back represents one's support and structure in life. Lower back: insecurity, fear of lack of money or primal support.

	Middle: guilt, powerlessness, feelings of shame, low self-esteem, selfish-driven decisions.
	Upper back: lack of emotional support, fear of life and love, grief, betrayal.
Hip Ailments	For women, the hips can represent emotional saddlebags, where stored and unexpressed emotions attach. Women tend to be more open in the hips (as nature requires for childbirth) and generally their emotions fluctuate more than men's. Men typically are more rigid in the hips, often taking some time to open in this region.
Neck & Shoulder Ailments	The neck and shoulders are where the daily stress and tension reside in the body—the weight of the world is often referred to as being carried on the shoulders. The neck has the physical ability to restrict the direction in which we're looking, as reflected by mental confusion over which way to turn. The shoulder blades and upper back carry and support the heart. Restriction and pain through the shoulders can relate to heartache and betrayal, cautiousness in opening up and trusting others with one's heart. Through heartache and disappointment, one can make life a burden purely via one's attitude.

Prana and the Breath

Prana is the vital life-force energy, the vitality that animates every living organism on all levels: humans, animals, and plants. It is the intelligence that coordinates the senses and is the key to unveiling the higher states of consciousness. Prana heals and restores the body on a cellular and energetic level. Keep in mind it is on this subtle level that the physical ailments originate from - the mental and emotional afflictions.

Energy and matter bear an important connection. If energy is compressed or harnessed, matter is the result. Where matter is diffused, energy is the result. The breath is the energizing force governing the matter in our bodies. As the primary muscle influencing the breath, the diaphragm is metaphysically considered the bridge between the conscious and the unconscious. The breath is the most prominent mechanism for connecting the mind and the body, the conscious and the sub-conscious, leading us to the doorway of the 'observer's room' where inner dialogue is witnessed and the higher self / God / Brahma is above all heard. Note that the lungs tend to reflect one's ability to take in life, to invite the fresh, new change.

The breath is the main pranic vehicle. The other vehicles are food, water, and sunlight. The breath is the most the vital part of any yoga practice. Pranayama is referred to as control or regulation of the breath and thus of prana. To breathe consciously is to infuse the physical body with divine light, the vital force. The breath is our first action when entering this life and our last when we leave; we can survive days without food or water, but only minutes without the breath. Yogis consider that the breath and the higher consciousness are two sides of the same coin. For thousands of years yogis have been connecting, influencing, retaining, and deepening the breath through pranayama techniques in order to connect with the higher consciousness on a mental level, and transcend the emotions on a sentiment level, while maintaining the human body (the physical vehicle in this lifetime), in physical form.

The way that you feel is directly reflected in the way that you breathe. To alter the way you feel, consciously change the way you're breathing. By breathing slowly and deeply, you instantly relax the nervous system and increase the prana circulating in the body. As the diaphragm is stimulated, the nervous system transcends the emotions. Physically, it massages the kidney, liver, lungs, and heart. Through proper yogic breathing, you will ultimately obtain the maximum benefits during asana practice. You will enhance every asana physically, both internally and externally. Internally, the body's systems (digestive, nervous, endocrine, glandular, reproductive) are stimulated and balanced by the fresh oxygenated blood and prana flowing freely. Externally, you deepen and refine the posture; inhaling to elongate the spine, thus the sushumna (refer to definition below) while softening and surrendering into the asana. Conscious breathing equals a quiet, calm mind. Therefore, by breathing consciously throughout the asana practice, you surpass the mind chatter, bringing about a tranquil state and finding further endurance. That endurance in turn takes us back to where the internal and external physical benefits can be truly achieved. One can practice the same asana a thousand times and always experience a deeper, more beautiful level, both physically and mentally, if the breath is conscious; we are peeling the many layers of an onion.

When prana is blocked in the body, toxins and stagnant waste accumulate; the body becomes stiff and restricted; and so too does the mind. As your yoga practice evolves, you will become more attentive to prana, enhancing and directing its flow. The mind and body become invigorated, as the prana restores and revitalizes the body on a cellular level; inevitably your inner awareness begins to expand and your intuition sharpens.

Chakras and Nadis

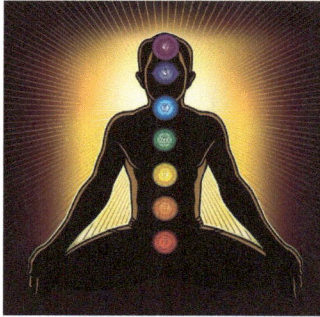

The concept of chakras and nadis originates from Hindu text dating to thousands of years ago, and features in yogic traditions of Hinduism and Buddhism. Chakras are energy centers or energy wheels in the human body; each chakra corresponds to different glands and governs specific parts of the physical body and areas of the psyche. Chakras draw in the divine life-force energy, the prana, and distribute this vital energy to the physical glands and organs throughout the body and bloodstream specific to achieving optimum health, well-being, and spiritual evolution. Chakras are considered to be interrelated and to affect one another; therefore, achieving optimum balance of the chakras provides a state of total emotional and physical well-being. When our chakras are balanced, maximum vitality and health is experienced. Physical or emotional trauma, along with negative thinking, will affect the corresponding chakra. Hatha yoga is one of many ways that distributes prana through all of the chakras, cleansing and balancing them.

The Seven Major Chakras

1. Root Chakra (Mooladhara)
   Associated with: Survival / Primal Instincts, Energetic foundation, Vitality, Strength, Money, Security, Karma
   Demon: Fear
2. Sacral Chakra (Swadhisthana)
   Associated with: Sacred Self, Emotional Body, Creativity, Sexual Energy

Demon: Guilt
3. Solar Plexus (Manipura)
   Associated with: Power Center, Self-Esteem, Willpower
   Demon: Shame
4. Heart Chakra (Anahata)
   Associated with: Compassion, Love, Harmony, Trust; Also
   the meeting point of the physical and spiritual bodies
   Demon: Grief
5. Throat Chakra (Vishuddhi)
   Associated with: Communication, Honesty, Self-Expression
   Demon: Dishonesty
6. Third Eye Chakra (Ajna)
   Associated with: Intuition, Emotional Intellect, Inner -
   Wisdom
   Demon: Illusion
7. Crown Chakra (Sahasrara)
   Associated with: Awareness, Spiritual Awakening;
   Connection to higher consciousness and awareness of the
   ego self
   Demon: Attachment

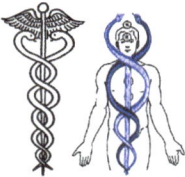

Nadis
Prana infuses the whole body, following flow patterns called nadis,
enabling the body to move and the mind to think. 'Nadi' literally
means 'flow' or 'current'; nadis are the subtle channels through
which the prana flows. Although there are thousands of nadis
within the subtle body, the three main nadis discussed here are ida,
pingala, and sushumna.

Sushumna runs in line with the spine, and ida and pingala commence at the root chakra crisscrossing and intercepting at each chakra (as represented by the snakes in the above diagram).

"When ida and pingala nadis are purified and balanced, and the mind is controlled, then sushumna, the most important nadi, begins to flow." *Asana, Pranayama, Mudra, Bandha* by Swami Satyanadanda Saraswati (1969)

The main intention of Hatha yoga is to bring about a balanced flow of prana through the ida and pingala nadis. Once sushumna begins to flow, this in turn awakens the kundalini energy— the potential spiritual energy that lies dormant, coiled like a snake in the Root Chakra. Therefore, the practice of asanas regulates and purifies the nadis, while stimulating the chakras, which in turn distributes the kundalini energy generated throughout the entire body and being.

'Ha' literally translates to 'sun' while 'tha' means 'moon'; representing the polar opposites, ying and yang, masculine / feminine. The current that is flowing at any given time can be recognized in the nostrils; one nostril is always more flared then the other and when the flow is equal between the two, sushumna is predominant. The right nostril 'ha' represents the sun energy or the masculine, while the left nostril 'tha' represents the lunar energy or feminine.

Nadi Shodhana (Alternate Nostril Breathing)
When looking to generate heat and energy in the body, focus on the sun energy by breathing consciously only through the right nostril. Physically, the right nostril corresponds to the left side of the brain, representing the masculine energy; when this pathway is clear, so too is the ability to think logically and practically. Conversely, the left nostril embodies the feminine, lunar energy. When looking to relax the body, focus on breathing consciously through only the left nostril. When this pathway is clear, so too is one's intuition and creativity. If the mind is overactive through

meditation, this is a sign that ida is imbalanced.

In order to balance both ida and pingala nadis, practice Nadi Shodhana (alternate nostril breathing) which is considered to clear the channels. Find a comfortable seated position, rest the left hand on the left knee in jana mudra (index finger curled with the tip of the thumb touching) and bring the right hand to the forehead. Place the index finger on the third eye center, curl the middle and ring fingers to the palm, and use the thumb and little finger to block alternate nostrils. To begin, block the right nostril with the thumb, inhale through the left nostril, hold the breath, then block the left nostril with the little finger and exhale through the right nostril, pause, then inhale through the right nostril and exhale through the left. Continue for as long as comfortable and when the practice begins to flow then apply mula bandha on the inhalation and release the bandha on the exhalation. On completion exhale through the left nostril last then relax the right hand down to the knee, inhale through both nostrils while applying mula bandha, pause, then exhale when needed, relax, and soften.

Yoga Nidra

Yoga Nidra is also known as yogic sleep or psychic sleep. It is an essential tool for complete rejuvenation. In normal sleep, the consciousness mind is absent and the unconscious mind is in charge. In Yoga Nidra the conscious mind directs the unconscious to relax, thus harmonizing the two hemispheres of the brain and the two aspects of the autonomous nervous system (sympathetic and parasympathetic). A blissful state of awareness is achieved as tension, stress, and the resultant blocked energy are released.

Through the deep, relaxed state Yoga Nidra induces, one is able to influence the subconscious mind in order to manifest one's goals. An essential feature of Yoga Nidra is the 'Sankalpa' also known as a positive affirmation or resolve. This is your personal goal which you program into the subconscious mind. Yoga Nidra induces alpha-level brain waves; the truly relaxed mind and body are perfect soil to plant your Sankalpa, the seed of your personal goal. The affirmation is short, positive, and precise about what you would like to achieve.
Examples: I am peaceful, I am achieving total health, I am awakening my spiritual potential

Your Sankalpa should never influence another's personal will.

An effective Yoga Nidra is said to be equivalent to four hours of sleep!

ABOUT THE AUTHOR

Nicole's personal practice began to evolve in the early 1990s. She is now a senior Yoga Teacher, has also studied in the metaphysical field, and is Reiki attuned.

Yoga is a beautiful journey, a valuable and an essential tool, a blessing in this life.

Om Shanti

www.ingramcontent.com/pod-product-compliance
Lightning Source LLC
Chambersburg PA
CBHW041223270326
41933CB00001B/21